AF492917

Table of Contents

How to Boost Your Immune System — The Neuropathic Way 5

What Is Immune System? 6

Immune System Diseases 10

Immune System Boosters........................... 12

1. Echinacea 13

2. Elderberry 15

3. Astragalus Root 16

4. Ginseng 18

Foods 20

5. Bone Broth.. 20

6. Ginger 21

7. Green Tea............................. 23

8. Vitamin C Foods 23

9. Beta-Carotene Foods 25

10. Probiotics 27

11. Vitamin D 29

12. Zinc 30

Essential Oils 31

13. Myrrh............................... 31

14. Oregano............................ 32

Lifestyle 34

15. Exercise 34

16. Reduce Stress...................... 35

17. Improve Sleep 36

18. Limit Alcohol Consumption 37

19. Take Protective Measures 38

Risk and Side Effects 38

12 Naturopathic Ways To Help Boost Your Immune

System 40

The Benefits of Natural Remedies for Seniors 41

Final Thoughts 52

How to Boost Your Immune System — The Neuropathic Way

We are continually exposed to organisms that are inhaled, swallowed or inhabit our skin and mucous membranes. Whether or not these organisms lead to disease is decided by the integrity of our body's defense mechanisms, or immune system.

When our immune system is working properly, we don't even notice it. But when we have an under- or over-active immune system, we are at a greater risk of developing infections and other health conditions.

If you are wondering how to boost your immune system, be advised that it doesn't necessarily happen over night. It's a matter of strengthening your immune response with lifestyle changes and the use of immune-boosting antimicrobial and antiviral herbs. But hopefully you find comfort in knowing that your body is made to combat germs and protect your body from harm.

What Is Immune System?

The immune system is an interactive network of organs, white blood cells and proteins that protect the body from viruses and bacteria or any foreign substances.

The immune system works to neutralize and remove pathogens like bacteria, viruses, parasites or fungi that enter the body, recognize and neutralize harmful substances from the environment, and fight against the body's own cells that have changes due to an illness.

Our immune system works to protect us every day, and we don't even notice it. But when the performance of our immune system is compromised, that's when we face illness. Research indicates that underactivity of the immune system can result in severe infections and tumors of immunodeficiency, while overactivity

results in allergic and autoimmune diseases.

For our body's natural defenses to run smoothly,

the immune system must be able to differentiate

between "self" and "non-self" cells, organisms and

substances. Here's a breakdown of the differences:

"Non-self" substances are called antigens, which

includes the proteins on the surfaces of bacteria,

fungi and viruses. Cells of the immune system

detect the presence of antigens and work to

defend themselves.

"Self" substances are proteins on the surface of our own cells. Normally, the immune system has already learned at an earlier stage to identify these cells proteins as "self," but when it identifies its own body as "non-self," and fights it, this is called an autoimmune reaction.

The amazing thing about the immune system is that it's constantly adapting and learning so that the body can fight against bacteria or viruses that change over time. There are two parts of the immune system:

Our innate immune system works as a general defense against pathogens.

Our adaptive immune system targets very specific pathogens that the body has already has contact with.

These two immune systems complement each other in any reaction to a pathogen or harmful substance.

Immune System Diseases

Before learning exactly how to boost your immune system, first understand that most immune disorders result from either an excessive immune response or an autoimmune attack. Disorders of the immune system include:

Allergies and Asthma

Allergies are a immune-mediated inflammatory response to normally harmless environmental substances known as allergens. The body overreacts to an allergen, causing an immune reaction and allergy symptoms. This can result in one or more allergic diseases such as asthma, allergic rhinitis, atopic dermatitis and food allergies.

Immune Deficiency Diseases

An immune deficiency disease is when the immune system is missing one or more of its parts, and it reacts too slowly to a threat. Immune deficiency conditions, like HIV/AIDS and drug-induced immune deficiency, are due to a severe impairment of the immune system, which leads to infections that are sometimes life-threatening.

Autoimmune Diseases

Autoimmune diseases cause your immune system to attack your own body's cells and tissues in response to an unknown trigger. Examples of autoimmune diseases include rheumatoid arthritis, lupus, inflammatory bowel disease, multiple sclerosis and type 1 diabetes.

Immune System Boosters

When searching for how to boost your immune system, look to these herbs, foods, supplements, essential oils and lifestyle factors.

Herbs

1. Echinacea

Many of echinacea's chemical constituents are powerful immune system stimulants that can provide significant therapeutic value. Research shows that one of the most significant echinacea benefits is its effects when used on recurring infections.

A 2012 study published in Evidence-Based Complementary and Alternative Medicine found that echinacea showed maximal effects on recurrent infections, and preventive effects increased when participants used echinacea to prevent the common cold.

A 2003 study conducted at the University of Wisconsin Medical School found that echinacea demonstrates significant immunomodulatory activities. After reviewing several dozen human experiments, including a number of blind randomized trials, researchers indicate that echinacea has several benefits, including immunostimulation, especially in the treatment of acute upper respiratory infection.

2. Elderberry

The berries and flowers of the elder plant have been used as medicine for thousands of years. Even Hippocrates, the "father of medicine," understood that this plant was key for how to boost your immune system. He used elderberry because of its wide array of health benefits, including its ability to fight colds, the flu, allergies and inflammation.

Several studies indicate that elderberry has the power to boost the immune system, especially because it has proven to help treat the symptoms of the common cold and flu.

A study published in the Journal of International Medical Research shows that when elderberry was used within the first 48 hours of onset of symptoms, the extract reduced the duration of the flu, with symptoms being relieved on an average of four days earlier. Plus, the use of rescue medication was significantly less in those receiving elderberry extract compared with placebo.

3. Astragalus Root

Astragalus is a plant within the bean and legumes family that has a very long history as an immune system booster and disease fighter. Its root has been used as an adaptogen in Traditional Chinese Medicine for thousands of years. Although astragalus is one of the least studied immune-boosting herbs, there are some preclinical trials that show intriguing immune activity.

A recent review published in the American Journal of Chinese Medicine found that astragalus-based treatments have demonstrated significant improvement of the toxicity induced by drugs such as immunosuppressants and cancer chemotherapeutics.

Researchers concluded that astragalus extract has a beneficial effect on the immune system, and it protects the body from gastrointestinal inflammation and cancers.

4. Ginseng

The ginseng plant, belonging to the Panax genus, can help you to boost your immune system and fight infections. The roots, stems and leaves of ginseng have been used for maintaining immune homeostasis and enhancing resistance to illness or infection.

Ginseng improves the performance of your immune system by regulating each type of immune cell, including macrophages, natural killer cells, dendritic cells, T cells and B cells. It has also proven to possess antimicrobial compounds that work as a defense mechanism against bacterial and viral infections.

A study published in the American Journal of Chinese Medicine suggests that ginseng extract successfully induces antigen-specific antibody responses when it's administered orally. Antibodies bind to antigens, such as toxins or viruses, and keep them from contacting and harming normal cells of the body.

Because of ginseng's ability to play a role in antibody production, it helps the body to fight invading microorganisms or pathogenic antigens.

Foods

5. Bone Broth

Bone broth supports immune function by promoting the health of your gut and reducing inflammation caused by leaky gut syndrome. The collagen and amino acids (proline, glutamine and arginine) found in bone broth help to seal openings in the gut lining and support its integrity.

We know that gut health plays a major role in immune function, so consuming bone broth works as an excellent immune system booster food.

6. Ginger

Ayurvedic medicine has relied on ginger's ability for how to boost your immune system before recorded history. It's believed that ginger helps to break down the accumulation of toxins in our organs due to its warming effects. It's also known to cleanse the lymphatic system, our network of tissues and organs that help rid the body of toxins, waste and other unwanted materials.

Ginger root and ginger essential oil can treat a wide range of diseases with its immunonutrition and anti-inflammatory responses. Research shows that ginger has antimicrobial potential, which helps in treating infectious diseases.

It's also known for its ability to treat inflammatory disorders that are caused by infectious agents such as viruses, bacteria and parasites, as well as physical and chemical agents like heat, acid and cigarette smoke.

7. Green Tea

Studies evaluating the efficacy of green tea show that it contains antioxidant and immunomodulatory properties. It works as an antifungal and antivirus agent, and may be helpful for immunocompromised patients.

Strengthen your immune system by drinking a good-quality green tea daily. The antioxidants and amino acids present in this tea will help your body to fight germs and get well.

8. Vitamin C Foods

Vitamin C foods, like citrus fruits and red bell peppers, improve the health of your immune system by providing anti-inflammatory and antioxidant properties.

Studies display that getting enough vitamin C (along with zinc) in your diet may help to reduce the symptoms of respiratory infections and shorten the duration of illnesses like the common cold and bronchitis.

The best vitamin C foods to add for a strong immune system include:

citrus fruits, including orange, lemon and grapefruit

black currant

guava

green and red bell pepper

pineapple

mango

honeydew

parsley

9. Beta-Carotene Foods

Beta-carotene has powerful antioxidant activity, allowing it to help reduce inflammation and fight oxidative stress. Instead of taking beta-carotene supplements, researchers propose that beta-carotene can promote health when taken at dietary levels, by eating foods rich in the carotenoid.

The richest sources of beta-carotene are yellow, orange and red fruits and veggies, and leafy greens. Adding the following foods to your diet can help promote a strong immune system:

Carrot juice

pumpkin

sweet potato

red bell peppers

apricot

kale

spinach

collard greens

Supplements

10. Probiotics

Because leaky gut is a major cause of food sensitivities, autoimmune disease and immune imbalance or a weakened immune system, it's important to consume probiotic foods and supplements.

Probiotics are good bacteria that help you digest nutrients that boost the detoxification of your colon and support your immune system.

Research published in Critical Reviews in Food Science and Nutrition suggests that probiotic organisms may induce different cytokine responses. Supplementation of probiotics in infancy could help prevent immune-mediated diseases in childhood by improving the gut mucosal immune system and increasing the number of immunoglobulin cells and cytokine-producing cells in the intestines.

11. Vitamin D

Vitamin D can modulate the innate and adaptive immune responses and a vitamin D deficiency is associated with increased autoimmunity as well as an increased susceptibility to infection.

Research proves that vitamin D works to maintain tolerance and promote protective immunity. There have been multiple cross-sectional studies that associate lower levels of vitamin D with increased infection.

One study conducted at Massachusetts General Hospital included 19,000 participants, and it showed that individuals with lower vitamin D levels were more likely to report a recent upper respiratory tract infection than those with sufficient levels, even after adjusting for variables such as season, age, gender, body mass and race. Sometimes addressing a nutritional deficiency is how to boost your immune system.

12. Zinc

Zinc supplements are often used as an over-the-counter remedy for fighting colds and other illnesses. It may help to reduce cold-related symptoms and shorten the duration of the common cold.

Research evaluating the efficacy of zinc shows that it can interfere with a molecular process that causes bacteria buildup in the nasal passages.

Essential Oils

13. Myrrh

Myrrh is a resin, or sap-like substance, that is one of the most widely used essential oils in the world. Historically, myrrh was used to treat hay fever, clean and heal wounds and stop bleeding. Studies conclude that myrrh strengthens the immune system with its antiseptic, antibacterial and antifungal properties.

A 2012 study validated myrrh's enhanced antimicrobial efficacy when used in combination with frankincense oil against a selection of pathogens. Researchers expressed that myrrh oil has anti-infective properties and can help to boost your immune system.

14. Oregano

Oregano essential oil is known for its healing and immune-boosting properties. It fights infections naturally due to its antifungal, antibacterial, antiviral and anti-parasite compounds.

A 2016 study published in Critical Reviews in Food Science and Nutrition found that the main compounds in oregano that are responsible for its antimicrobial activity include carvacrol and thymol.

Several scientific studies show that oregano oil exhibited antibacterial activity against a number of bacterial isolates and species, including B. laterosporus and S. saprophyticus.

Lifestyle

15. Exercise

Incorporating physical activity into your daily and weekly regimen is extremely important to strengthen your immune system.

A 2018 human study published in Aging Cell revealed that high levels of physical activity and exercise improve the immunosenescence (gradual deterioration of the immune system) in older adults aged 55 through 79, compared to those in the same age group who were physically inactive.

The study also highlights that physical activity doesn't protect against all of the immunosenescence that occurs. However, the decrease in a person's immune system function and activity can be influenced by decreased physical activity in addition to age.

16. Reduce Stress

Studies prove that chronic stress can suppress protective immune responses and exacerbate pathological immune responses.

In order to promote health and healing, you need to minimize your stress levels. This can be difficult today, especially when people are concerned about becoming ill, but it's important.

17. Improve Sleep

When you aren't getting enough sleep, your immune system won't be able to function properly. In fact, research analyzing the vulnerability of sleep-deprived adults found that those who slept less than six hours a night were more than four times likely to get a cold than adults who slept more than seven hours.

To reduce your chances of catching colds and the flu, make sure you're getting at least seven hours of sleep every night.

18. Limit Alcohol Consumption

Consuming too much alcohol can certainly impact immune function, which is why you'll need to cut back on alcohol to fight infections and promote immune system health.

Alcohol negatively impact gut health, decreasing immune function and making you more susceptible to harmful pathogens. Stick to one or 2 alcohol drinks a week, or less, to boost your immune system.

When there are germs and bugs going around, it's important to protect yourself and those around you. This means:

frequent hand washing, for at least 20 seconds

minimize touching your face

staying home when sick

coughing or sneezing into your elbow

seeking medical attention and treatment when needed

Risk and Side Effects

In the quest for how to boost your immune system, proceed with some caution. If you are using these immune-boosting herbs, supplements and essential oils, remember that the products are extremely potent and should not be taken for more than two weeks at a time. Giving yourself a break in between long doses is important.

Also, if you are pregnant, be cautious when using essential oils and reach out to your health care provider before doing so.

Any time you are using natural remedies like plant supplements, it's a good idea to do it under the care of your doctor or nutritionist.

12 Naturopathic Ways To Help Boost Your Immune System

When it's chilly and rainy outside, and cold and flu season is at its height, it's time to pull out all the stops to keep our families in good health and tiptop shape. Regular doctor visits and appropriate seasonal vaccines are, of course, a must. But when it comes to easing the sniffles and preventing illness on a day-to-day basis, many of us turn to the content of our medicine cabinets — or our kitchens. However, there are several natural treatments that not only help us feel better, but have also been proven to help boost the immune system.

The Benefits of Natural Remedies for Seniors

Those of us with senior loved ones are well aware that dietary needs, physical abilities and immunity itself all change with age. The immune response tends to get weaker, making vaccines less effective and infections more likely. Diet — specifically, getting the right nutrients — is one of the keys to maintaining immune health, but there are numerous other little steps we can take at home to boost immunity in ourselves and our families.

Herbal teas, dietary supplements and even some types of gentle exercise like tai chi fall under the category of naturopathy, or naturopathic medicine. Using therapies both traditional and modern, "Practitioners view their role as supporting the body's ability to maintain and restore health, and prefer to use treatment approaches they consider to be the most natural and least invasive," says the NIH's National Center for Complementary and Integrative Health. Introduced with care and attention, naturopathic remedies can empower us to take charge of our own health and help us boost our immune systems to prevent illness and promote well-being.

Remember that consultation with a qualified physician is always the best route to take before implementing any major changes to the daily routine, particularly with herbal medicines or other dietary interventions that may have unexpected interactions with traditional medications.

According to Harvard Medical School, in order to function well, our immune systems require balance and harmony. Here are several ways to promote that balance through diet, exercise, supplements and other healthy-living strategies.

1. Remember your A-B-C-D-Es. A lack of micronutrients — i.e., vitamins — has been linked to reduced immunity. Taking a multivitamin supplement, along with eating a healthy diet rich in natural sources of nutrients, boosts overall health as well as the immune system. In particular, vitamins A, B2, B6, C, D and E have been studied in relation to immune response, and seem to play a key role in helping us avoid illness.

2. Get some sun. Spending some time in natural light is one of the key ways our bodies manufacture vitamin D. Vitamin D plays a role in helping our immune systems produce antibodies;

low levels of vitamin D, on the other hand, have been correlated with a higher risk of respiratory infection.

3. Open your mouth and say "om." While the physical effects of stress are still being studied by scientists, studies have so far proven that chronic stress can lead to a variety of negative effects on physical and emotional well-being, including a reduced immune response. Stress-reducing practices like meditation, massage, and even music can help us relax and improve our immune function.

4. Try turmeric. The bright orange-yellow spice that gives curries a distinct flavor and mustard its color also has anti-inflammatory properties, and there is increasing evidence that it helps prevent illness, too. Particularly relevant for seniors, extracts of turmeric seem to play a role in preventing cancer, slowing Alzheimer's, and alleviating arthritis pain.

5. Run a relaxing bath. A nice hot bath, with Epsom salt or relaxing aromatherapy scents, can go a long way toward reducing our stress — and making us sleepy. Sleep is one of the key ways our bodies repair themselves, and sleep deprivation, reports

Mother Earth News, "activates the stress response, depresses immune function and elevates inflammatory chemicals."

6. Eat more vegetables. Vegetables, as well as fruits, nuts, and seeds, are loaded with nutrients that we need to keep our immune systems in top health. In particular, cruciferous vegetables like cabbage, kale, and broccoli help support liver function, a key part of our bodies' natural detoxification process.

7. Micromanage your minerals. In addition to a range of vitamins, it is important to get enough —

but not too much — of key minerals that are important to daily health. Selenium, according to Harvard Medical School, may help prevent cancer, and zinc is a critical ingredient for the proper function of our immune cells. However, experts caution that too much zinc can actually impair immune function, so it's important to stick to the recommended daily allowance.

8. Make room for 'shrooms. Certain types of mushrooms, particularly Japanese mushrooms like shiitake, maitake, and oyster mushrooms, have recently been shown to help support the

production of immune cells. They're also loaded with antioxidants.

9. Try herbal remedies. Scientists are still studying the effectiveness of many herbal supplements traditionally used as health boosters, like echinacea and ginseng, but whether or not they have a measurable effect on the immune system, a soothing tea can help with relaxation, sleep, and stress reduction. Of course, you should always talk to a doctor before making herbal treatments a regular part of your arsenal.

10. Spice up your cooking. Pungent but tasty garlic and ginger are both delicious, immune-boosting additions to the family diet. Raw garlic in particular contains antimicrobial and cancer-fighting agents, and ginger has been used for centuries in traditional medicine to treat nausea, colds, and flu symptoms.

11. Keep on moving. Regular exercise contributes to our overall health in numerous ways, and a healthy body means a smoothly functioning immune system. Some forms of exercise, like tai chi and yoga, are also particularly suited for reducing stress and improving the strength,

balance and flexibility that we often lose as we age.

12. Consider taking probiotics. Probiotics, or "good" bacteria, are not only an important part of a healthy digestive process but also our immune systems, though scientists are still studying exactly how and why this happens. A study on athletes found that probiotic supplements helped prevent and combat colds, but you can also get probiotics from naturally fermented food sources, like yogurt and kimchi.

Boosting your family's immunity doesn't have to be a chore — in fact, it can be delicious, relaxing, and fun. Just make sure to consult a doctor before beginning any major changes to your regimen, and don't forget those medical tests and flu shots, especially for senior loved ones.

Final Thoughts

The immune system is an interactive network of organs, cells and proteins that protect the body from viruses and bacteria or any foreign substances.

When the immune system is working properly, you don't even notice it. It's when the performance of the immune system is compromised that you face

illness.

Plants, herbs, minerals, foods and lifestyle changes

can be used to prevent and fight infections due to

their   antimicrobial   and   immune-boosting

properties.

Home treatments and natural remedies can help

us take charge of our day-to-day health and boost

immunity during the season of colds, the flu and

sniffles.